Keto Meat & Soup Slow Cooker Cookbook

The Complete Soup and Meat cookbook for your keto slow cooker diet; 50 easy and delicious recipes!

Lilith Wolfe

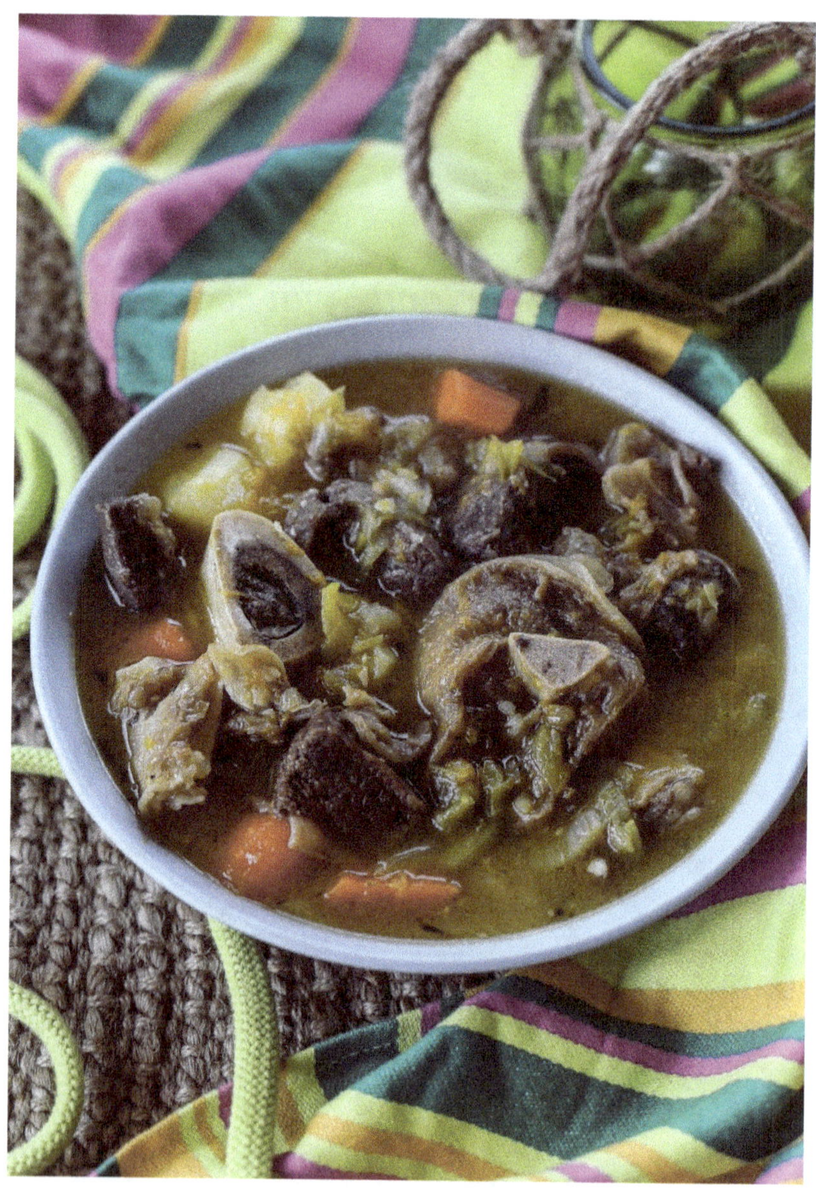

indirectly. Respective authors own all copyrights not held by the publisher.

The information herein is offered for informational purposes solely and is universal as so. The presentation of the information is without contract or any type of guarantee assurance.

Table of contents

Slow Cooker Cheeseburger Soup

Preparation time: 15 minutes

Cooking time: 3 hours

Servings: 5

Ingredients:

1/2 tsp salt

1/2 tsp pepper

1/2 cup cheese

1/2 cup chopped onions

1/2 chopped red bell pepper

1 tsp garlic powder

1 tsp Worcestershire sauce

1 1/2 tsp parsley

1 1/2 chopped tomatoes

1 1/2 pounds ground beef

2 chopped & cooked bacon slices

3 cups beef broth

3 chopped celery sticks

8 ounces tomato paste

Directions:

Using a large saucepan, add in the ground beef and brown.

Halfway through the browning process, drain off every fat, add in the red pepper, onions, celery, and continue cooking.

Add the remaining **Ingredients** and beef mixture into the crockpot then stir to combine.

If desired, add in more beef broth, cover, and cook for 6-8 hours on low setting or 3-5 hours on a high setting, occasionally stirring.

Serve then top with a full spoon of cheese and bacon slices (if desired), then enjoy.

Nutrition:

Calories: 200 Carbs: 14g

Fat: 13g Protein: 7g

Chicken Thigh & Breast Low Carb Soup

Preparation time: 5 minutes

Cooking time: 6 hours

Servings: 6

Ingredients:

1/2 tsp fresh ground pepper

1 tsp sea salt

1 chopped medium onion

1 tsp apple cider vinegar

1 tbsp. herbs de Provence

2 organic skin on & bone chicken thighs

2 organic skin on & bone-in chicken breasts

3 diced carrot s

3 diced celery stalks

3-4 cups filtered water

Directions:

Place the **Ingredients** in layers inside the crockpot.

Make sure the bone side of the chicken is down on top of the veggies.

Add in surplus water until the veggies are submerged, and the chicken is covered halfway.

Cover the crockpot then cook for 6-8 hours.

Remove the chicken from the crockpot one done and cool, then remove the bones and skin.

Shred the chicken, then return into the crockpot, season to taste, reheat, then serve and enjoy.

Nutrition:

Calories: 97

Carbs: 6g

Fat: 2g

Protein: 14g

Beef & Pumpkin Stew

Preparation time: 5 minutes

Cooking time: 4 hours

Servings: 4

Ingredients:

1 teaspoon sage

1 teaspoon mixed herbs

2 tablespoons rosemary

2 tablespoons thyme

6 tablespoons coconut oil

200g pumpkin

300g stewing steak

salt & pepper, to taste

Directions:

Trim off every excess fat from the stewing steak then transfer it into the crockpot.

Season the steak with half of the coconut oil then and in the salt & pepper.

Cover the crockpot then cook on high setting for 1 hour.

Remove the steak from the crockpot to a serving platter alongside all the remaining seasoning and coconut oil.

Mix everything, then transfer back into the crockpot with the pumpkin and cook for 3 hours on a low setting. Serve with the fresh mixed herbs and enjoy.

Nutrition:

Calories: 324 Carbs: 37g

Fat: 11g Protein: 23g

Pepper Jalapeno Low Carb Soup

Preparation time: 10 minutes

Cooking time: 7 hours

Servings: 8

Ingredients:

1/4 tsp paprika

1/2 tsp pepper

1/2 chopped onion

1/2 tsp xanthan gum

1/2 chopped green pepper

1/2 cup heavy whipping cream

1/2 lb. cooked & crumbled bacon

3/4 cup cheddar Cheese

3/4 cup Monterrey Jack Cheese

1 tsp salt

1 tsp cumin

1 & ½-pounds chicken breasts, boneless

2 minced garlic cloves

2 seeded & chopped jalapenos

3 tbsps. butter

3 cups chicken broth

6 oz. cream cheese

Directions:

Dissolve the butter, then cook the green peppers, seasoning, jalapenos, and onions until translucent in a medium-sized pan.

Scoop the mixture into the crockpot, then add in the chicken broth and breast.

Cover the crockpot then cook for 3-4 hours on high or 6-7 hours on a low setting.

Separate the chicken, and shred it, then return it into the crockpot.

Put in the heavy whipping cream, cream cheese, remaining cheeses, bacon then stir until the cheese melts.

Sprinkle the soup with xantham gum to thicken, then allow it to simmer uncovered on low for 10 minutes.

Serve, then top with cheddar cheese, bacon, or jalapenos and enjoy.

Nutrition:

Calories: 240 Carbs: 1g

Lean Beef & Mixed Veggies Soup

Preparation time: 8 minutes

Cooking time: 6 hours

Servings: 6

Ingredients:

1/2 tsp garlic salt, if desired

1 peeled small onion

1 diced small green pepper

1 tsp garlic & herb seasoning

1 small zucchini, sliced into rounds

1 can rinse & drained cannellini beans

1 small yellow squash, sliced into rounds

1 (14 1/2 ounces) can diced roasted tomatoes

1 & ½-pounds beef stew meat

1-2 tsp ground pepper

1-3 bay leaves

2 cups of frozen mixed vegetables

4 cups low salt beef broth

4 peeled & chopped garlic cloves

Directions:

Add all the **Ingredients** except the zucchini cannellini beans, mixed vegetables, and yellow squash into the crockpot.

Cover the pot then cook on high for 4 hours.

After 4 hours, add in the zucchini, cannellini beans, yellow squash, and mixed vegetables .

Season to taste, and cook for an extra 2 hours on high.

Once done, stir then serve and enjoy.

Nutrition:

Calories: 50 Carbs: 10g

Fat: 0g Protein: 2g

Chicken & Tortilla Soup

Preparation time: 7 minutes

Cooking time: 2 hours & 10 minutes

Servings: 6

Ingredients:

1 diced sweet onion

1 teaspoon cumin

1 teaspoon chili powder

1 neatly chopped cilantro bunch

1 (28 ounces) can diced tomatoes

1-2 cups water

2 cups celery, chopped

2 cups carrots, shredded

2 tablespoons tomato paste

2 diced & de-seeded jalapenos

2 big skinned chicken breasts, sliced into 1/2" strips

4 minced garlic cloves

32 ounces organic chicken broth

olive oil

sea salt & fresh cracked pepper, as desired

Directions:

Pour a dash of olive oil, 1/4 cup of chicken broth, the garlic, onions, pepper, jalapeno, and sea salt into a Dutch oven and cook over medium-high heat until soft.

Transfer the mixture into the crockpot and ass in the remaining **Ingredients** and cook for 2 hours on low settings.

Shred the chicken, then top with the cilantro, avocado slices and enjoy.

Nutrition:

Calories: 130

Carbs: 16g

Fat: 5g

Protein: 8g

Chicken Chile Verde

Preparation time: 12 minutes

Cooking time: 6 hours

Servings: 9

Ingredients:

1/4 teaspoon sea salt

2 pounds chopped boneless chicken.

3 tablespoons divided butter

3 tablespoons neatly chopped & divided cilantro

5 minced & divided garlic cloves

1 extra tablespoon cilantro, to garnish

1 1/2 cups salsa Verde

Directions:

Dissolve 2 tablespoons butter in the slow cooker on high.

Add in 4 of the garlic along with 2 tablespoons cilantro then stir.

Use a stovetop, melt 1 tablespoon butter in a big frypan over medium-high heat, and add 1 tablespoon minced garlic and cilantro.

Put in the chopped chicken, then sear until all the sides are browned but not cooked through.

Add the cilantro, garlic, and butter mixture with browned chicken into the crockpot.

Pour in the salsa Verde and stir together.

Cover the crockpot and cook on high settings for 2 hours, then reduce to a low setting for 3-4 extra hours.

Serve the chicken Verde in a lettuce cup or over cauliflower rice.

Nutrition:

Calories: 140

Carbs: 6g

Fat: 4g

Protein: 18g

Cauliflower & Ham Potato Stew

Preparation time: 5 minutes

Cooking time: 4 hours

Servings: 6

Ingredients:

1/4 tsp salt

1/4 cup heavy cream

1/2 tsp onion powder

1/2 tsp garlic powder

3 cups diced ham

4 garlic cloves

8 oz. grated cheddar cheese

14 1/2 oz. chicken broth

16 oz. bag frozen cauliflower florets

a dash peppers

Directions:

Put all the items except the cauliflower inside the crockpot and mix.

Cover the crockpot then cook for 4 hours on high setting.

Once done, add in the cauliflower and cook for an extra 30 minutes on high. Serve and enjoy.

Nutrition:

Calories: 71

Carbs: 2g

Fat: 4g

Protein: 6g

Minestrone Ground Beef Soup

Preparation time: 15 minutes

Cooking time: 8 hours

Servings: 1

Ingredients:

1/2 tsp basil, dried

1/2 tsp oregano, dried

1/2 cup vegetable broth

1 diced carrot

1 lb. ground beef

1 diced yellow onion

1 diced celery stalk

1 tbsp. garlic, minced

1 (28 ounces) can diced tomatoes

2 diced small zucchini

Directions:

Using a medium-sized pan on a stovetop, place in the ground beef and brown.

Boil 3 cups of water. Transfer the boiled water and browned beef into the crockpot Put in the remaining fixing into the crockpot.

Cook for 5-8 hours on low settings. Serve and enjoy.

Nutrition:

Calories: 180 Carbs: 24g

Fat: 4g Protein: 13g

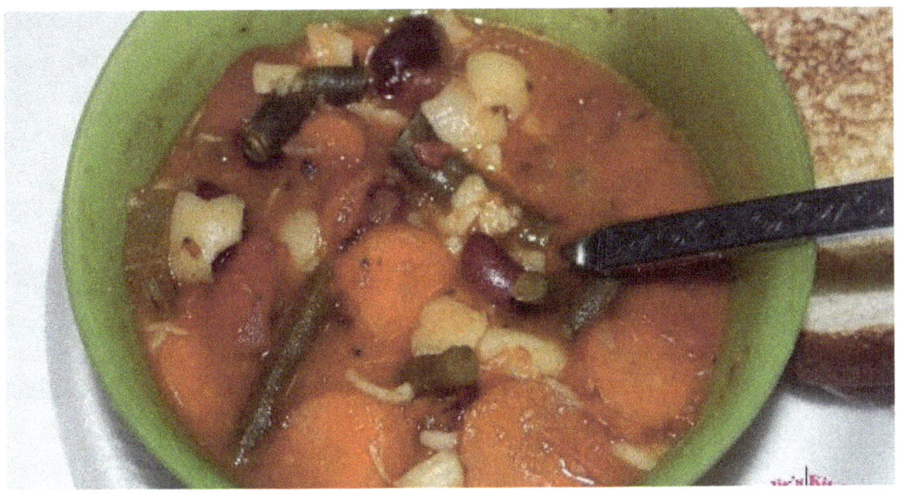

Scrumptious Crab Meat Douse

Preparation time: 15 minutes

Cooking time: 5 hours

Servings: 5

Ingredients:

1 package Vegetable recipe mix

1 container sour cream

1 package cream cheese, softened

1 teaspoon lemon juice

1 can crab meat, thawed and drained

Directions:

Put all your fixing into your slow cooker and cook on low heat settings for 4-5 hours. Toss together before serving.

Nutrition:

Calories: 110 Carbs: 1g

Fat: 9g

Protein: 6g

Slow Cooker Bay Carrot Garlic Beef Sauce

Preparation time: 20 minutes

Cooking time: 12 hours

Servings: 6

Ingredients:

4 carrots, chopped

1 bay leaf

2 pounds beef stew meat, slice

1 teaspoon paprika

1 stalk celery, diced

1/4 cup all-purpose flour

1 teaspoon Worcestershire sauce

1/2 teaspoon salt

3 potatoes, diced

1 clove garlic, shredded

1 onion, diced

1/2 teaspoon ground black pepper

1 1/2 cups beef broth

Directions:

Mix your salt, flour, and pepper in a small bowl.

Put your beef in the crockpot and pour your flour mixture on it.

Toss together to coat beef.

Put all the other items inside the crockpot and stir together.

Cover and cook on low heat settings for 11-12 hours.

Nutrition:

Calories: 159

Carbs: 20g

Fat: 6g

Protein: 2g

Delicious Kernel Corn Taco Soup

Preparation time: 10 minutes

Cooking time: 8 hours

Servings: 8

Ingredients:

1 package taco seasoning mix

1-pound ground beef

1 can whole kernel corn, with liquid

1 onion, chopped

1 can dice green chili peppers

1 can tomato sauce

2 cans peeled and diced tomatoes

1 can chili beans, with liquid

2 cups of water

1 can kidney beans with liquid

Directions:

Sauté your beef in a skillet until it is brown on all sides and keep aside.

Put your browned beef into your crockpot and add all other **Ingredients** and toss together to blend evenly.

Cook within 8 hours, low.

Nutrition:

Calories: 83

Carbs: 14g

Fat: 3g

Protein: 1g

Sumptuous Ham and Lentil Consommé

Preparation time: 15 minutes

Cooking time: 11 hours

Servings: 6

Ingredients:

8 teaspoons tomato sauce

1 cup onion, diced

1 cup dried lentils

1 cup of water

1 cup celery, chopped

1/2 teaspoon dried basil

32 ounces chicken broth

1 cup carrots, diced

1/4 teaspoon dried thyme

1/4 teaspoon black pepper

2 cloves garlic, minced

1/2 teaspoon dried oregano

1 1/2 cups diced cooked ham

1 bay leaf

Directions:

Put all your fixing into your slow cooker and mix very well to blend well.

Cook within 11 hours, low heat settings. Remove your bay leaf before serving it.

Nutrition:

Calories: 194

Carbs: 21g

Fat: 4g

Protein: 20 g

Beef Barley Vegetable Soup

Preparation time: 15 minutes

Cooking time: 8 hours

Servings: 10

Ingredients:

1 package frozen mixed vegetables

Ground black pepper to taste

1 beef chuck roast

1 onion, chopped

salt to taste

1/2 cup barley

4 cups of water

1 can chop stewed tomatoes

1 bay leaf

3 stalks celery, chopped

1/4 teaspoon ground black pepper

3 carrots, chopped

4 cubes beef bouillon cube

2 tablespoons oil

1 tablespoon white sugar

Directions:

Season your beef with salt, adding bay leaf and barley in the last hour; cook your beef in your slow cooker for 8 hours or until tender.

Set your beef aside; keep your broth also aside.

Stir fry your onion, celery, carrots, and frozen vegetable mix until soft.

Add your bouillon cubes, pepper, water, salt, beef mixture, barley mixture, chopped stewed tomatoes, and broth.

Bring to boiling point and simmer at lowered heat for 20 minutes.

Nutrition:

Calories: 69

Carbs: 10g

Fat: 2g

Protein: 5g

Delicious Chicken Soup with Lemongrass

Preparation time: 5 minutes

Cooking time: 8 hours

Servings: 10

Ingredients:

1 stalk of lemongrass, cut into big hunks

1 whole chicken

1 Tablespoon of salt

5 thick slices of fresh ginger

20 fresh basil leaves (10 -slow cooker; 10 -spices)

1 lime

Directions:

Put your lemongrass, ginger, 10 basil leaves, salt, and chicken into the slow cooker.

Fill the slow cooker up with water. Boil the chicken mixture for 480 - 600 minutes.

Scoop the soup into a bowl and adjust your salt to taste. Juice in the lime to taste and spice up with the chopped basil leaves.

Nutrition:

Calories: 105

Carbs: 1g

Fat: 2g

Protein: 15g

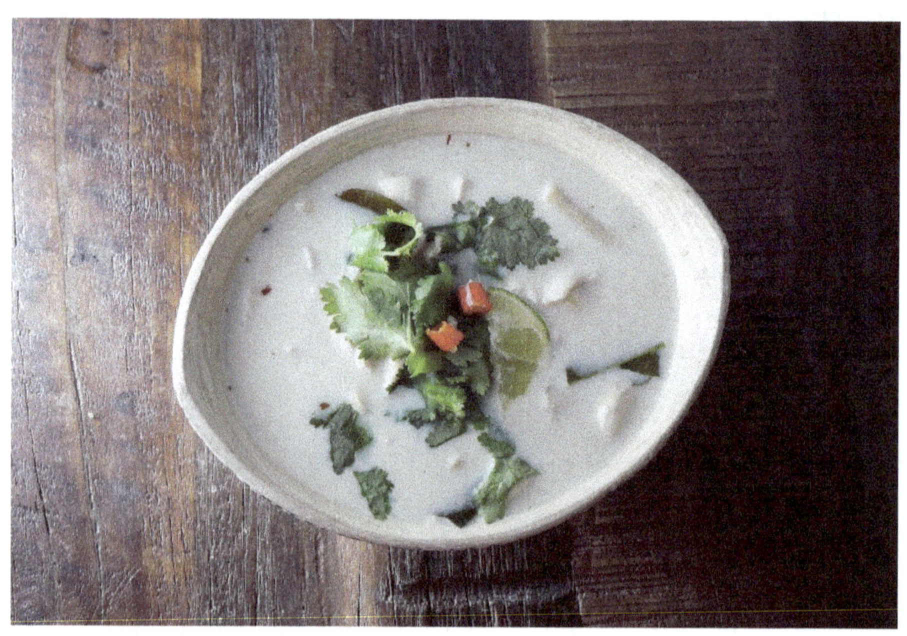

Slow Cooker Pork Stew with Tapioca

Preparation time: 15 minutes

Cooking time: 10 hours

Servings: 6

Ingredients:

3 tablespoons quick-cooking tapioca

1 tablespoon vegetable oil

1/4 teaspoon pepper

1 large onion, chopped

1 1/2 lb. pork stew meat, cut into bite-size pieces

2 teaspoons Worcestershire sauce

1 stalk celery, chopped

4 carrots, sliced

1 tablespoon beef bouillon granules

3 red potatoes, cubes

3 cups vegetable juice

Directions:

Heat your oil over medium-high heat using a Dutch oven; brown your beef on all sides.

Mix your browned beef with all other **Ingredients** in the crockpot.

Cover and cook on low heat settings for 9-10 hours.

Nutrition:

Calories: 190 Carbs: 0g

Fat: 10g

Protein: 23g

Delicious Bacon Cheese Potato Soup

Preparation time: 15 minutes

Cooking time: 10 hours

Servings: 8

Ingredients:

3 lb. large baking potatoes, peeled, cut into 1/2-inch cubes

1/4 cup chopped fresh chives

8 slices bacon, diced

1 carton fat-free reduced-sodium chicken broth, divided

1/2 cup milk

1 onion, finely chopped

1 pkg. Shredded Triple Cheddar Cheese, divided

1/2 cup Sour Cream

2 tablespoons flour

Directions:

Stir fry bacon over medium heat in a large skillet. Remove bacon with your slotted spoon and leave the drippings in the skillet.

Stir fry your onions in the skillet for few minutes until it is soft and crisp. Add in your flour and cook for 1 minute, stirring it frequently.

Add 1 cup of your chicken broth and cook for 2-3 minutes or until sauce is thick and simmers. Pour the sauce into your slow cooker

.

Add your remaining chicken broth and potatoes and cook with slow cooker cover for 8-10 hours on low heat settings.

Transfer 4 cups of your potatoes in a bowl and mash it until smooth, adding 1.5 cups of cheese to the remaining mixture in the slow cooker; stir until melted.

Stir your mashed potatoes into the slow cooker with milk added and cook again within 5 minutes with the lid.

Microwave your bacon in a microwavable plate within 30 seconds or until heated.

Serve your soup with bacon, using sour cream, chives, and remaining cheese as toppings.

Nutrition:

Calories: 100

Carbs: 18g

Fat: 0g

Protein: 2g

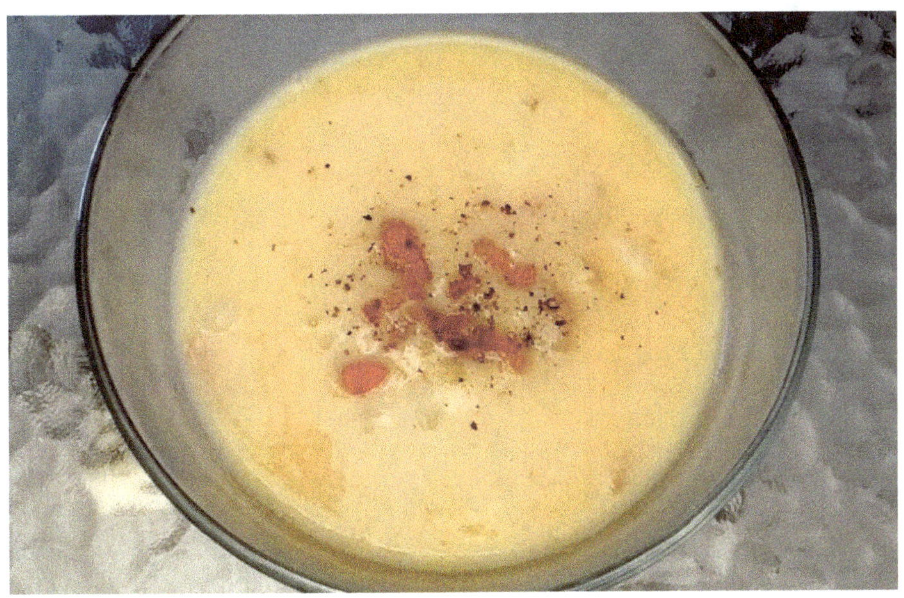

Tasty Tomato Soup with Parmesan and Basil

Preparation time: 15 minutes

Cooking time: 3 hours

Servings: 6

Ingredients:

28 oz of tomatoes, chopped

1/2 cup heavy cream

1/2 cup grated Parmesan cheese

10-12 large basil leaves

3 tablespoons chopped garlic

2-3 **Servings** of Erythritol

1/2 tablespoon dried thyme

1/4 teaspoon of red pepper flakes

1 tablespoon onion powder

Directions:

Add all **Ingredients** except your parmesan and heavy cream to your crockpot and cook on high heat for 3 hours.

Add your cheese and cream and stir. Adjust seasoning to taste. Enjoy

Nutrition:

Calories: 110

Carbs: 16g

Fat: 3g

Protein: 5g

Luscious Carrot Beef Stew with Potatoes

Preparation time: 15 minutes

Cooking time: 10 hours

Servings: 8

Ingredients:

32 oz beef broth

One teaspoon oregano

2 cups baby carrots

2 pounds beef stew meat, bite-sized

2 celery ribs, chopped

1 tablespoon dried parsley

¼ cup of water

1 tsp Salt

1 cup of frozen corn

2 Tablespoons Worcestershire sauce

2-3 cloves of garlic, grated

¼ cup flour

6oz can tomato paste

1 tsp pepper

4-5 red potatoes, bite-sized

1 cup frozen pea

1 medium onion, finely chopped

Directions:

Add your tomato paste, beef, beef broth, celery, Worcestershire sauce, carrots, oregano, red onions, parsley, potatoes, garlic, salt, and pepper into your crockpot and mix.

Cook on low heat for 10 hours.

Mix the flour plus water in a small bowl and pour it into your crockpot 30 minutes before serving and mix until well combined.

Stir in your corn and frozen peas and cook for another 30 minutes in the crockpot, covered.

Nutrition:

Calories: 262

Carbs: 9g

Fat: 10g

Protein: 20g

Delicious Lasagna Consommé

Preparation time: 15 minutes

Cooking time: 7 hours

Servings: 8

Ingredients:

2 cups uncooked shell pasta

1 tablespoon dried parsley

1 can of diced tomatoes

1 cup of water

3 cups of beef broth

¼ teaspoon pepper

1 tablespoon dried basil

¼ teaspoon salt

½ cup chopped onion

1 cup V8

4-5 cloves of garlic, grated

1, 6oz can of tomato paste

1 lb. ground beef

Shredded cheese- topping

Directions:

Mix your tomato pastes and can tomatoes in your crockpot.

Add your garlic, salt, broth, V8, pepper, basil, beef, and parsley.

Mix, then cook on low heat for 7 hours.

Precisely 30 minutes left of **Cooking time**, add 1 cup of water and noodles into your crockpot. Stir together and cook with the lid back on for 30 minutes.

Nutrition:

Calories: 68

Carbs: 5g

Fat: 0g

Protein: 12g

Sumptuous Cheese Broccoli Potato Bouillabaisse

Preparation time: 15 minutes

Cooking time: 8 hours

Servings: 8

Ingredients:

1 tablespoon butter

1 1/2 lbs. potatoes, chopped into 3/4 in cube s

2 1/2 cups boiling water

1 cup onion, sliced

1 package frozen broccoli, chopped

1 package cheddar cheese, minced

2 chicken bouillon cubes

Directions:

Butter the saucepan and fry your onions until crisp.

Add your water, bouillon cubes, sautéed onions, and potatoes into a pot and cover it up. Cook under medium heat until potatoes are soft.

Place your cheddar cheese and broccoli in your crockpot while you cook your potatoes. Melt and defrost your cheese and broccoli on low heat settings.

Blend your soft potatoes contents using a food processor to your desired consistency and pour it into your crockpot.

Heat up on low heat settings until it is warm.

Nutrition:

Calories: 240

Carbs: 5g

Fat: 9g

Protein: 34g

Balsamic Beef Pot Roast

Preparation time: 30 minutes

Cooking time: 3 hours

Servings: 10

Ingredients:

1 boneless (3 lb.) chuck roast

1 tbsp. of each:

Kosher salt

Black ground pepper

Garlic powder

¼ c. balsamic vinegar

½ c. chopped onion

2 c. water

¼ t. xanthan gum

For the Garnish: Fresh parsley

Directions:

Massage the chuck roast with garlic powder, pepper, plus salt over the entire surface. Use a large skillet to sear the roast until browned.

Deglaze the bottom of the pot using balsamic vinegar—Cook one minute. Add to the slow cooker.

Mix in the onion, and add the water. Once it starts to boil, secure the lid, and continue cooking on low for three to four hours.

Remove the meat, then chopped it into large chunks. Remove all fat and anything else that may not be healthy such as too much fat.

Mix the xanthan gum into the broth, then put it back to the slow cooker.

Serve and enjoy with a smile!

Nutrition:

Calories: 393

Carbs: 3 g

Protein: 30 g

Fat: 28 g

Beef Bourguignon with Carrot Noodles

Preparation time: 20 minutes

Cooking time: 5 hours

Servings: 6

Ingredients:

5 slices - thick-cut bacon

1 (3 lb.) chuck roast/round roast/your favorite

1 large yellow onion

3 diced celery stalks

1 bay leaf

3 large minced garlic cloves

4 sprigs of fresh thyme

1 lb. sliced white button mushrooms

1 tbsp. tomato paste

1 c. of each:

-Beef/chicken broth (+) more as needed

-Red wine

1 large/2 med. carrots

For the Garnish: Chopped parsley

Salt & Pepper

Optional: Dash of red pepper flakes

Directions:

Prepare the bacon in a frying pan using the medium-high on the stovetop. Drain the grease. Put pepper and salt to taste in the meat cubes. Set the meat in the skillet, cook 1 to 3 minutes, then turn it over and cook for about 2 minutes each side. Put in the slow cooker once the cubes are cooked. Fold in the pancetta, garlic, mushrooms, celery, and onion in the cooker. Push the thyme and bay leaves between the layers.

Empty the porridge and wine to cover the batter within ¾ of the way up the cooker.

Cook for 4 hours on high setting. Make the carrots into a 'noodle' using a peeler. Cook again within an hour.

Trash the bay leaves when the meal is done and mix well. Serve with the parsley and pepper flakes.

Nutrition:

Calories: 548 Carbs: 6 g

Fat: 32 g Protein: 50 g

Beef Brisket

Preparation time: 20 minutes

Cooking time: 8 hours

Servings: 6

Ingredients:

1 (3-4 lb.) brisket

2 t. smoked of each:

Salt

Paprika

1 t. of each:

Onion powder

Black pepper

Garlic powder

Directions:

Towel-dry the brisket and mix the spices with rubbing the meat before placing it in the slow cooker. Put the brisket, then cook about eight hours on the low setting.

Warm up the oven to 150°F.

Put the brisket in a broiler-safe pan, then keep it in the oven while you prepare the gravy. Strain the cooking liquids into a jar.

Place the skimmed cooking juices in a medium saucepan to simmer over medium heat. Whisk until you reach a creamy sauce, usually about 10 minutes.

Transfer the brisket onto a cutting surface and cover loosely with foil to keep it warm. Rest it within 10 minutes, then cut the brisket into slices going against the grain. Put the sauce over the top and serve enjoy.

Nutrition:

Calories: 582 Carbs: 0 g

Fat: 44 g Protein: 42 g

Beef Curry

Preparation time: 35 minutes

Cooking time: 5 hours

Servings: 8

Ingredients:

2 ½ lb. chuck roast

6 tbsp. coconut milk powder

2 c. water

3 tbsp. red curry paste

5 cracked cardamom pods

2 tbsp. of each:

Dried Thai chilis/fresh red chilis

Thai fish sauce

1/8 teaspoon of each:

Cloves

Nutmeg

1 tbsp. of each:

Dried onion flakes

Ground coriander

Ground ginger

ground cumin

Granulated sugar substitute

Serving **Ingredients**:

2 tbsp. of each:

Coconut milk powder

Granulated sugar substitute

1 tbsp. red curry paste

¼ c. chopped of each:

Fresh cilantro

Cashews (can omit)

Optional: ¼ t. xanthan gum

Directions:

Arrange the chuck roast in the cooker. Empty the milk, water, fish sauce, curry paste, ginger, cloves, nutmeg, coriander, cumin, your chosen sweetener, the onion flakes, chilis, and cardamom pods. Secure the top of the pot. Use the low setting for eight hours or high for five hours.

Right before serving, arrange the meat on a plate.

Whisk the sauce with two tablespoons of the milk powder, the xanthan gum, sugar substitute sweetener, and curry paste. Tear the meat to shreds, and stir into the sauce. Garnish with some cilantro, and serve.

Nutrition:

Calories: 351 Protein: 26.0 g

Carbs: 5 g Fat: 22 g

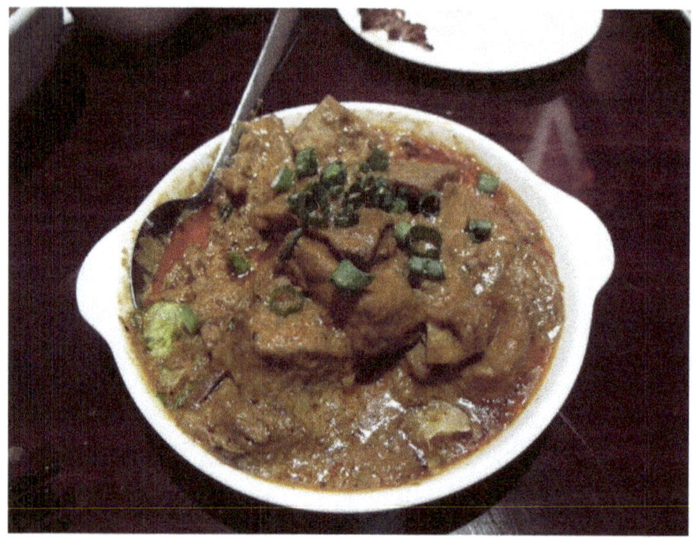

Beef Dijon

Preparation time: 15 minutes

Cooking time: 5 hours

Servings: 4

Ingredients:

4 (6 oz.) small round steaks

2 tbsp. of each:

Steak seasoning - to taste

Avocado oil

Peanut oil

Balsamic vinegar/dry sherry

4 tbsp. large chopped green onions/small chopped onions for the garnish - extra

1/4 c. whipping cream

1 c. fresh crimini mushrooms - sliced

1 tbsp. Dijon mustard

Directions:

Warm up the oils using the high heat setting on the stovetop. Flavor each of the steaks with pepper and arrange to a skillet. Cook two to three minutes per side until done.

Place into the slow cooker. Pour in the skillet drippings, half of the mushrooms, and the onions.

Cook within 4 hours, low.

When the **Cooking time** is done, scoop out the onions, mushrooms, and steaks to a serving platter.

Whisk the mustard, balsamic vinegar, whipping cream, and the steak drippings from the slow cooker.

Empty the gravy into a gravy server and pour over the steaks. Enjoy with some brown rice, riced cauliflower, or potatoes.

Nutrition:

Calories: 535

Carbs: 5.0 g

Fat: 40 g

Protein: 39 g

Beef Ribs

Preparation time: 30 minutes

Cooking time: 6 hours

Servings: 4

Ingredients:

3 lb. beef back ribs

1 tbsp. of each:

-Sesame oil

- Rice vinegar

- Hot sauce

- Honey

- Garlic powder

- Kosher salt

½ t. black pepper

1 tbsp. potato starch/ cornstarch

¼ c. light soy sauce/ coconut aminos

Directions:

Arrange the ribs in your slow cooker. Cut them in half if it doesn't fit well in your cooker.

Whisk the rest of the **Ingredients** together, but omit the cornstarch for now.

Put the sauce batter over the ribs, set to low, then cook within 6 hours. It will be fall off the bone tender.

Prepare the oven to 200°F.

Transfer the ribs to a baking pan, and cover with foil to keep warm.

Strain the liquid into a saucepan, then set to high setting, then mix in the cornstarch with cold water .

Continue cooking within five to ten minutes. Put the glaze sauce over the ribs, then serve.

Nutrition:

Calories: 342 Carbs: 7 g

Fat: 27 g

Protein: 23 g

Beef Stroganoff

Preparation time: 10 minutes

Cooking time: 6 hours

Servings: 10

Ingredients:

4 minced garlic cloves

1 c. white mushrooms (approx. 10)

1 large chopped onion

3 tbsp. chopped parsley

2 c. bone broth – homemade or Kettle & Fire (ex.)

2 lbs. beef roast into small strips

Pepper & salt to taste

Ingredients for Serving:

1 cucumber – peeled into long wide strips

½ c. coconut milk/cream

3 tbsp. Dijon mustard

Garnish with parsley

Salt to taste

Directions:

Arrange the strips of roast in the cooker. Stir in the salt, pepper, beef broth, mushrooms, garlic, and onion.

Cook for six to eight hours using the low-temperature setting.

When done, stir in the coconut cream, mustard, and salt.

Cover a serving bowl with the cucumber noodles.

Top it off with the stroganoff. Garnish with the parsley if desired.

Nutrition:

Calories: 462

Carbs: 4.0 g

Fat: 36 g

Protein: 26.0 g

Cabbage & Corned Beef

Preparation time: 10 minutes

Cooking time: 8 hours

Servings: 10

Ingredients:

6 lb. corned beef

1 large head of cabbage

4 c. water

1 celery bunch

1 small onion

4 carrots

½ t. of each:

Ground mustard

Ground coriander

Ground marjoram

Black pepper

Salt

Ground thyme

Allspice

Directions:

Dice the carrots, onions, and celery and toss them into the cooker. Pour in the water.

Combine the spices, rub the beef, and arrange in the cooker. Cook on low within seven hours.

Remove the top layer of cabbage. Wash and cut it into quarters it until ready to cook. When the beef is done, add the cabbage, and cook for one hour on the low setting. Serve and enjoy.

Nutrition:

Calories: 583

Carbs: 13 g

Fat: 40 g

Protein: 42 g

Chipotle Barbacoa – Mexican Barbecue

Preparation time: 10 minutes

Cooking time: 4 hours

Servings: 9

Ingredients:

½ c. beef/chicken broth

2 med. chilis in adobo (with the sauce, it's about 4 teaspoons)

3 lb. chuck roast/beef brisket

5 minced garlic cloves

2 tbsp. of each:

Lime juice

Apple cider vinegar

2 t. of each:

Sea salt

Cumin

1 tbsp. dried oregano

1 t. black pepper

2 whole bay leaves

Optional: ½ t. ground cloves

Directions:

Mix the chilis in the sauce, and add the broth, garlic, ground cloves, pepper, cumin, salt, vinegar, and lime juice in a blender, mixing until smooth.

Chop the beef into two-inch chunks, and toss it in the slow cooker. Empty the puree on top. Toss in the two bay leaves.

Cook four to six hours on the high setting or eight to ten using the low set.

Dispose of the bay leaves when the meat is done.

Shred the meat, then mix into the juices to simmer for five to ten minutes.

Nutrition:

Calories: 242

Carbs: 2 g

Fat: 11 g

Protein: 32 g

Corned Beef Cabbage Rolls

Preparation time: 25 minutes

Cooking time: 6 hours

Servings: 5

Ingredients:

3 ½ lb. corned beef

15 large savoy cabbage leave s

¼ c. of each:

White wine

Coffee

1 large lemon

1 med. sliced onion

1 tbsp. of each:

Rendered bacon fat

Erythritol

Yellow mustard

2 t. of each:

Kosher salt

Worcestershire sauce

¼ t. of each:

Cloves

Allspice

1 large bay leaf

1 t. of each:

Mustard seeds

Whole peppercorns

½ t. red pepper flakes

Directions:

Add the liquids, spices, and corned beef into the cooker. Cook six hours on the low setting.

Prepare a pot of boiling water. When the time is up, add the leaves and the sliced onion to the water for two to three minutes. Transfer the leaves to a cold-water bath - blanching them for three to four minutes. Continue boiling the onion.

Pat-dry the leaves. Put the onions plus beef, then roll up the cabbage leaves.

Drizzle with freshly squeezed lemon juice.

Nutrition:

Calories: 481.4

Carbs: 4.2 g

Protein: 34.87 g

Fat: 25.38 g

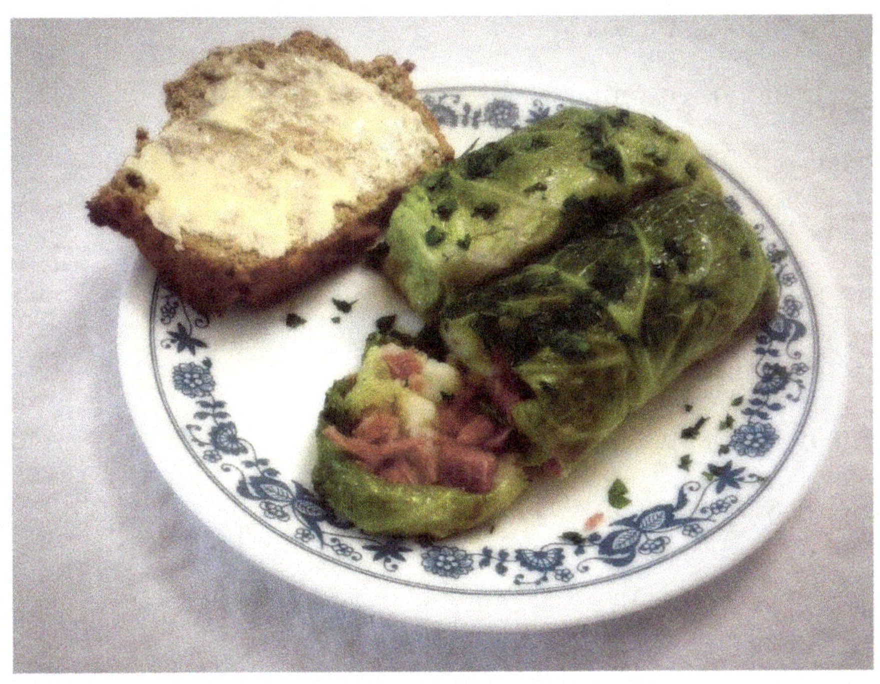

Cube Steak

Preparation time: 15 minutes

Cooking time: 8 hours

Servings: 8

Ingredients:

8 cubed steaks (28 oz.)

1 ¾ t. adobo seasoning/garlic salt

1 can (8 oz.) tomato sauce

1 c. water

Black pepper to taste

½ med. onion

1 small red pepper

1/3 c. green pitted olives (+) 2 tbsp. brine

Directions:

Slice the peppers and onions into ¼-inch strips.

Sprinkle the steaks with the pepper and garlic salt as needed and place it in the cooker.

Fold in the peppers, onion, water, sauce, and olives with the liquid/brine from the jar.

Close the lid. Prepare using the low-temperature setting for eight hours.

Nutrition:

Calories: 154

Carbs: 4 g

Protein: 23.5 g

Fat: 5.5 g

Eggplant & Ground Beef Casserole

Preparation time: 15 minutes

Cooking time: 4 hours

Servings: 12

Ingredients:

2 c. cubed eggplant

2 lb. ground beef

½ t. pepper

1 tbsp. olive oil

2 t. of each:

Salt

Mustard

Worcestershire sauce

1 can of each:

28 oz. drained diced tomatoes

16 oz. canned tomato sauce

1 t. oregano

2 c. grated mozzarella cheese

2 tbsp. parsley

Needed for the Slow Cooker: 9x13 pan

Directions:

Dust the salt over the cubed eggplant. Let it rest for 30 minutes. Add to a container and cover with the oil.

Mix the beef, salt, pepper, mustard, and Worcestershire sauce, then mash the mixture into the pan's bottom. Top it off with the eggplant, then spread out the tomatoes and sauce. Add in along with the rest of the fixings. Prepare using the high setting for two to three hours or low for three to four hours.

Nutrition:

Calories: 209 Protein: 15.9 g

Fat: 12.8 g Carbs: 5.7 g

Italian Meatballs & Zoodles

Preparation time: 35 minutes

Cooking time: 6 hours

Servings: 12

Ingredients:

1 medium spiraled zucchini

32. oz. beef stock

1 small diced onion

2 chopped celery ribs

1 chopped carrot

1 med. diced tomato

6 minced garlic cloves

1 ½ lb. ground beef

1 ½ t. garlic salt

½ c. shredded parmesan cheese

1 large egg

½ t. black pepper

4 tbsp. freshly chopped parsle y

1 ½ t. of each:

Onion powder

Sea salt

1 t. of each:

Italian seasoning

Dried oregano

Directions:

Warm up the slow cooker with the low setting function.

Add the zucchini, beef stock, onion, celery, tomato, garlic salt, and carrot to the cooker. Cover with the lid.

Combine the beef, egg, parmesan, parsley, Italian seasonings, pepper, sea salt, oregano, garlic, and onion powder in a mixing container. Mix and shape into 30 meatballs.

Warm up the oil using med-high heat in a frying pan. When it's hot, add the meatballs—Brown and toss it into the cooker.

Prepare with the lid on for six hours on the low setting.

Nutrition:

Calories: 129

Carbs: 3 g

Fats: 6 g

Protein: 15 g

London Broil

Preparation time: 20 minutes

Cooking time: 4 hours

Servings: 4

Ingredients:

2 LB. London broil

1 tbsp. Dijon mustard

2 tbsp. of each:

Reduced sugar ketchup

Coconut Aminos or soy sauce

½ c. of each:

Coffee

Chicken broth

¼ c. white wine

2 t. of each:

Onion powder

Minced garlic

Directions:

Arrange the beef in the slow cooker. Cover both sides with the mustard, soy sauce, ketchup, and minced garlic.

Pour the liquids into the cooker and give it a sprinkle of the onion powder.

Cook for four to six hours. When it's ready, shred the meat. Combine with the juices.

Serve and enjoy.

Nutrition:

Calories: 409

Carbs: 2.6 g

Fat: 18.3 g

Protein: 47.3 g

Machaca - Mexican Pot Roast

Preparation time: 20 minutes

Cooking time: 7 hours

Servings: 10

Ingredients:

3 ½ LB. beef chuck roast

2 t. granulated garlic

½ t. ground coriander

1 t. ground cumin

3 tbsp. bacon grease

1 t. freshly ground black pepper

Kosher salt

2 tbsp. of each:

Organic tomato paste

Worcestershire sauce

1 c. low-sodium beef/bone broth

2 c. fresh salsa

Directions:

Combine the garlic, cumin, salt, pepper, coriander, and cumin. Rub the beef all over.

Render the bacon grease in a large skillet using the med-high setting. Brown the meat (2 min. each side). Arrange in the slow cooker and add the salsa, Worcestershire, tomato paste, and broth over the roast. Add the juices from the bacon and cover the slow cooker.

Cook one hour on the high setting. Lower the heat and cook until tender on the low power setting – about six to eight hours.

When ready, shred, and remove any fat.

Place the meat back into the juices of the slow cooker. Stir to coat and serve.

Nutrition:

Calories: 365

Carbs: 3 g

Fat: 26 g

Protein: 27 g

Parmesan Garlic Nut Chicken Wings

Preparation time: 15 minutes

Cooking time: 4 hours

Servings: 4

Ingredients:

½ cup chicken wings

1/2 tablespoon chopped garlic

1 tablespoon olive oil

2 tablespoons ghee

1 tablespoon mayonnaise

1 tablespoon Stevia

1 tablespoon grated Parmesan cheese

1 teaspoon lemon juice

1 teaspoon apple cider vinegar

1 pinch of dry oregano

1 pinch of dried basil

Salt, pepper, and chili pepper to taste

Fresh basil or parsley (to embellish)

1 pinch xanthan gum optional thickener

Directions:

Mix all the items except for the chicken to make the sauce in a large bowl.

Smear the Slow Cooker with a little butter or a non-sticking spray, then pour half the sauce on the bottom. Add the chicken wings and cover .

Cook at HIGH temperature for 4 hours.

Take the chicken wings on a baking tray covering with aluminum foil.

Pour the left-over sauce on the wings and bake in the oven on grill mode for another 15 minutes at about 200 degrees C to get a crunchy crust.

Serve the chicken wings topped with garlic and parmesan while it's still hot.

Nutrition:

Calories: 180 Carbs: 1g

Fat: 16g Protein: 8g

Tikka Masala Chicken

Preparation time: 15 minutes

Cooking time: 4 hours

Servings: 4

Ingredients:

½ cup of chicken breast

2 tablespoons tomato sauce

2 tablespoons coconut milk

1 teaspoon fresh ginger

1 teaspoon thickener Xanatum gum

2 tablespoons olive oil

1 tablespoon cocoa butter

1 tablespoon of garam masala

1 pinch of cumin powder

1 pinch of Curcuma

1 pinch of ground black pepper

1 pinch of paprika

1 pinch of fresh coriander

1 dash of lemon juice

Directions:

Rinse the chicken breast leaving the skin and cut it into cubes of about 3 cm

With your hands, grease the chicken cubes all around in the cocoa butter so to soften the meat uniformly

Clean and chop the garlic and ginger. Regarding the ginger, you can also leave it in bigger pieces and remove it at the end of the cooking if you do not wish to eat it, otherwise chop it finely

Combine all spices and salt

At this point, combine all the **Ingredients** into the Slow Cooker, with the chicken and cover with tomato sauce, coconut milk, olive oil, and lemon juice. Stir well for the whole to season the meat evenly. Cook in the slow cooker within 4 hours, high.

Put a tablespoon of thickener, 1 hour before it's done, to thicken the cooking broth, and stir well to avoid lumps.

Garnish it all with crushed fresh coriander.

Nutrition:

Calories: 180 Carbs: 4g

Fat: 7g Protein: 25

Hot Spicy Chicken

Preparation time: 15 minutes

Cooking time: 3 hours

Servings: 5

Ingredients:

½ cup chicken, skinless

2 tablespoons olive oil

1 tablespoon fresh ginger root

1 tablespoon white onion, sliced

1 tablespoon cocoa butter

1 teaspoon rosemary needles

1 pinch of salt

Directions:

Cut the onion in slices, and roll it with your hands into the cocoa butter to soften.

Clean and divide the ginger into 2 parts. Put all the items in the slow cooker, adding salt and rosemary.

Cover it with oil, and mix the **Ingredients** well.

Cook in the slow cooker within 3 hours, high. After half of the **Cooking time**, turn the chicken over.

After cooking, pour over the chicken a bit of the stew liquid. The chicken will be uniquely soft.

Nutrition:

Calories: 140

Carbs: 10g Fat: 5g

Protein: 16g

Savory Duck Breast

Preparation time: 15 minutes

Cooking time: 5 hours

Servings: 6

Ingredients:

½ cup duck breast

2 tablespoons pine nuts

1 tablespoon fresh plums, diced

2 tablespoons carrot, diced

1 pinch of onion powder

2 tablespoons celery stalk, diced

2 tablespoons ghee

1 pinch of fresh basil, chopped

1 pinch of chili powder

1 pinch of salt

For the dip:

2 tablespoons / 28 gr of mayonnaise

1 pinch of chili powder

Directions:

Open the duck breast by placing the inside upward, season with salt and pepper and a dash of oil

Chop all the vegetables together and mix with the pine nuts, ghee, and plums, then put it on the Slow Cooker.

If you have a grid, put it in the pot over the vegetables and lay on it the duck.

Cook within 5 hours, high .

When finished cooking, remove the chest from the pot and place it on a plate, remove the skin that should be easily removable at this point

At this point, you can use the seasoning and pour it over the meat. Garnish with some basil leaves

Nutrition:

Calories: 180 Carbs: 0g

Fat: 6g Protein: 29g

Lemon Scented Chicken

Preparation time: 15 minutes

Cooking time: 4 hours

Servings: 3

Ingredients:

½ cup of chicken breast

2 tablespoons lemon juice

2 tablespoons of olive oil

1 pinch of rosemary, fresh

1 pinch of sage, fresh

1 pinch of garlic powder

1 oz of white wine (Pinot Grigio)

For the dip:

1 pinch of chili

1 tablespoon / 14 gr of eggplant, diced

2 tablespoons / 28 gr of mayonnaise

1 pinch of fresh parsley, chopped

1 pinch of garlic powder

1 dash of lemon juice

1 pinch of salt

Directions:

Put the chicken legs in a pan and sauté them with olive oil until each side becomes golden, sprinkling with white wine at the end.

Put the chicken into your Slow Cooker, add the lemon juice and a half lemon.

Add crushed herbs with garlic powder.

Add salt and cook on HIGH temperature for 4 hours.

In the meantime, prepare the dip. Preheat the oven to 480°F, then bake the eggplant for half an hour on a baking pan. Then remove and mix all of the dip **Ingredients** in a small bowl. Chill for a few hours to give the flavors time to develop

Nutrition:

Calories: 287 Carbs: 0g

Fat: 0g Protein: 0g

Autumn Sweet Chicken

Preparation time: 15 minutes

Cooking time: 5 hours

Servings: 6

Ingredients:

3 tablespoons Stevia powder

2 tablespoons walnuts, roasted

1 pinch of ground cinnamon

1 pinch of ground nutmeg

1 pinch of ground turmeric

A pinch of salt

1 boneless and skinless chicken leg

2 tablespoons olive oil

2 tablespoons ghee

1 pinch of onion powder

1 dash of lemon juice

1 oz of chicken broth

1 pinch of rosemary

½ cinnamon stick

Directions:

Roast the walnuts in a frying pan. Put it aside to cool.

Divide in half and use a blender to crumble half of them.

Mix the stevia, ground cinnamon, turmeric, nutmeg, and salt in a large bowl. Add the skinless chicken and roll it, so it is covered evenly.

Heat a frying pan and sauté the chicken until golden.

Dissolve the butter in the same pan on medium heat.

Put the onions powder, chopped nuts, lemon juice, and broth into your Slow Cooker pot with a spoon. Add the spicy chicken and the remaining spice mixture.

Add by mixing the garlic clove, rosemary, and cinnamon stick.

Cook within 5 hours, low.

Nutrition:

Calories: 454 Carbs: 53g

Fat: 15g

Protein: 30g

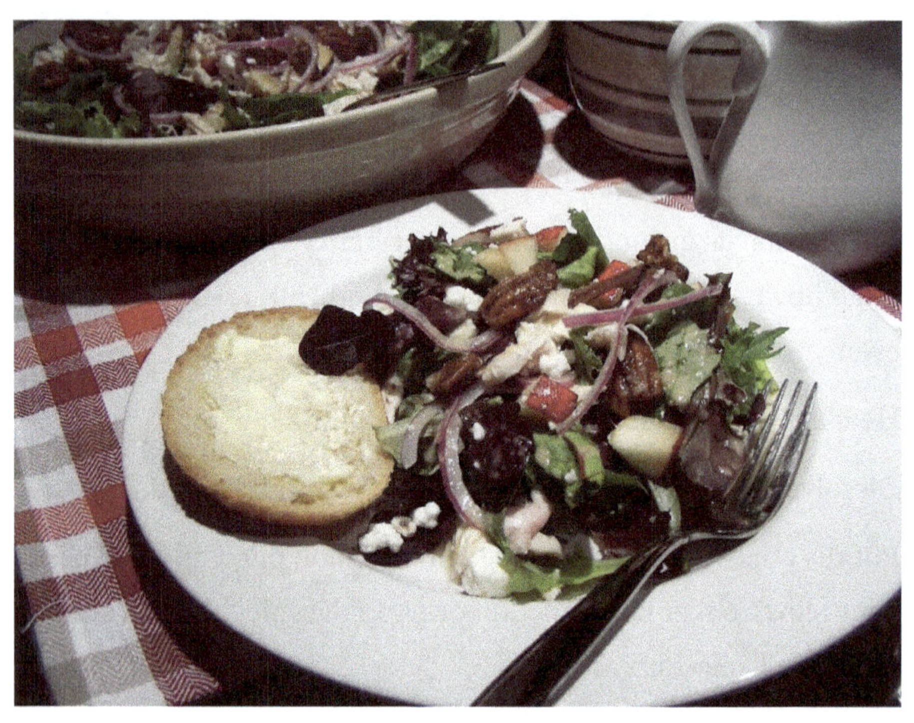

Coconut & Basil Chicken

Preparation time: 15 minutes

Cooking time: 4 hours

Servings: 4

Ingredients:

½ cup skinless and boneless chicken

1 oz of coconut milk

2 tablespoons ghee

1 tablespoon fresh basil leaves

1 teaspoon chopped ginger

1 clove garlic

1 dash of lime juice

1 pinch of cumin

For the dip:

2 tablespoons of olive oil

1 tablespoon grated coconut, dehydrated

1 pinch of curry

1 pinch of salt

1 pinch of fresh basil, chopped

Directions:

Prepare the chicken sauce combining the coconut milk, basil, ginger, garlic, lime juice, cumin, curry, salt, pepper, and cinnamon in a mixer. Mix until it's well combined.

Meanwhile, mix all the dip **Ingredients** mixing well. Put aside to chill for a few hours, so the flavors enrich.

Lay the skinless and boneless chicken in the slow cooker. Pour the sauce over the chicken and cook for 4 hours on high .

When the chicken is tender and well-cooked, separate it from the sauce.

Pour the sauce into a saucepan and heat it on the stove for a few minutes to make it denser, before pouring over the chicken on a plate.

Nutrition:

Calories: 240 Carbs: 30g

Fat: 5g Protein: 178g

BBQ Dip Hot Chicken Wings

Preparation time: 15 minutes

Cooking time: 6 hours

Servings: 5

Ingredients:

Ingredients for the chicken:

¼ cup skinless and boneless chicken

2 tablespoons of butter

1 tablespoon BBQ sauce

1 pinch of parsley

1 pinch of salt and black pepper

Ingredients for the BBQ dip:

For the BBQ dip sauce:

1 tablespoon ketchup

2 tablespoons olive oil

1 tablespoon liquid Stevia

1 teaspoon apple cider vinegar

1 pinch of pepper

1 pinch of onion powder

1 dash of Worcestershire sauce

Directions:

Lay the chicken breast in your Slow cooker.

Pour the BBQ sauce over the chicken, cover and cook on low for 6 hours.

Cut the butter in small pieces and smear all the chicken with it, leave it to cook again in an hour on low, removing the lid.

Serve hot with the dip as a side dish.

Nutrition:

Calories: 180 Carbs: 7g Fat: 10g

Protein: 18g

Cheesy Chicken Pot

Preparation time: 15 minutes

Cooking time: 8 hours

Servings: 4

Ingredients:

¼ cup skinless and boneless chicken

2 tablespoons white onion, chopped

2 tablespoons carrots, finely chopped

1 tablespoon Cheddar cheese, diced

2 tablespoons ghee

1 pinch of oregano

1 pinch of time

1 tablespoon cocoa butter

¼ cup sour cream

Directions:

Pour all of your **Ingredients** in the Slow Cooker pot, except for the sour cream, cocoa butter, and cheddar and ghee. Cook within 8 hours, low, and pour the sour cream, cheddar, and ghee.

Cook for another half an hour without the lid.

Nutrition:

Calories: 242

Carbs: 8g

Fat: 10g

Protein: 27g

Beijing Chicken Soup

Preparation time: 15 minutes

Cooking time: 4 hours

Servings: 3

Ingredients:

¼ cup finely chopped chicken scallops

1 oz chicken broth

2 tablespoons shitake mushrooms, minced

1 tablespoon fresh grated ginger

2 tablespoons carrots, julienne cut

2 tablespoons ghee

2 tablespoons olive oil

1 pinch of garlic powder

1 heart of lemongrass stem, crushed

1 tablespoon spicy soy sauce

1 pinch of freshly chopped coriander

1 oz of water

1 pinch of salt

Directions:

Pour in your Slow Cooker the vegetables, chicken, minced mushrooms, ginger, and garlic. Add the water, broth, lemongrass, soy sauce, and coriander. Cook within 4 hours, low.

Nutrition:

Calories: 125 Carbs: 4g Fat: 8g Protein: 10g

Lamb Curry

Preparation time: 15 minutes

Cooking time: 3 hours

Servings: 4

Ingredients:

1 lb. diced lamb

6 oz fresh baby spinach

5 teaspoons curry powder

15-ounces marinara sauce, sugar-free

1/2 cup water

Directions:

Place a medium-sized skillet over medium heat, grease with oil, and add the diced lamb.

Stir in the curry powder and a pinch of salt, cook gently for 7 to 10 minutes, or golden brown.

Transfer the meat into a 4-quart slow-cooker.

Stir in the marinara sauce and the water, ensuring the meat is fully immersed in the liquid.

Cover and seal the slow-cooker, allowing the food to cook for 3 hours at a high heat setting.

Mix in the spinach leaves, then continue cooking for another half hour, or until the spinach is tender.

Serve warm with cauliflower rice.

Nutrition:

Calories: 310 Carbohydrates: 5 g

Fats: 17 g Protein: 33 g

Lamb and Green Beans

Preparation time: 15 minutes

Cooking time: 6 hours

Servings: 4

Ingredients:

3 lb. lamb leg, on the bone

6 cups fresh green beans, trimmed

4 cloves of garlic, peeled and sliced

2 tablespoons dried mint

2 cups of chicken broth or water

Directions:

Massage the lamb on all sides with salt and black pepper.

Place a large skillet over medium heat, allow 2 tablespoons of butter to melt, then add the seasoned lamb.

Allow to brown, frequently turning; to make it is golden brown on all sides. It should take 10 – 15 minutes.

Transfer the lamb to the slow-cooker, sprinkle with the garlic and mint, and add the water.

Cover the slow-cooker with the lid, and allow the lamb to cook for 6 hours at a high heat setting.

Check occasionally and if the lamb gets dry, pour in an additional 1/2 cup of water.

Place the beans into the slow-cooker, and allow to continue cooking for another hour. The beans should be tender-crisp.

Serve hot.

Nutrition:

Calories: 525

Carbohydrates: 12 g

Fats: 36.4 g

Protein: 37.3 g

Lamb Shoulder

Preparation time: 15 minutes

Cooking time: 7 hours

Servings: 4

Ingredients:

1 lamb shoulder, on the bone

2 tablespoons mixed herbs

1/4 teaspoon xanthan gum

2 cups chicken stock, warmed

Directions:

Grease a 4-quarts slow-cooker with a non-stick cooking spray.

Season the lamb with the mixed herbs and a pinch of salt and pepper, and place it in the slow-cooker.

Pour over the stock, and seal the slow-cooker with its lid. Cook within 7 to 8 hours, allow the meat to cook on a low heat setting, or until the meat is tender.

Transfer the lamb meat to a plate and keep warm.

Transfer the cooking liquid into a saucepan, stir in the xanthan gum and allow to cook gently until the gravy has reduced to the desired thickness.

Carve the meat into slices, and serve with a jug of gravy alongside.

Nutrition:

Calories: 488 Carbohydrates: 1 g

Fats: 36 g

Protein: 39 g

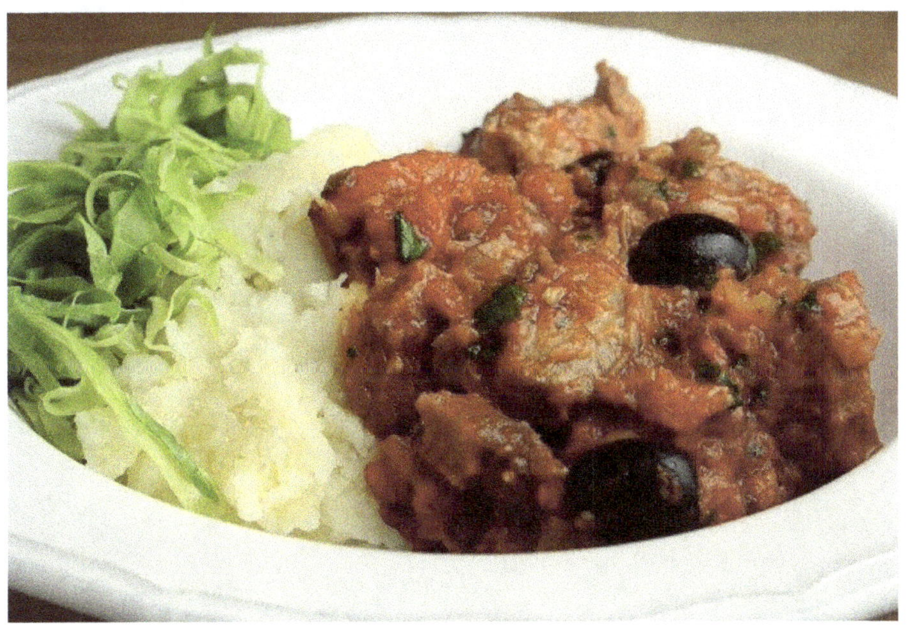